The Thyroid Diet Plan

───── ❧❧❧❧ ─────

How To Maximize Energy, Boost Metabolism and Maintain Healthy Hormone Levels

liable for any hardship or damages that may befall them after undertaking information described herein.

Additionally, the information in the following pages is intended only for informational purposes and should thus be thought of as universal. As befitting its nature, it is presented without assurance regarding its prolonged validity or interim quality. Trademarks that are mentioned are done without written consent and can in no way be considered an endorsement from the trademark holder.

Table of Contents

Introduction

Congratulations on downloading *The Thyroid Diet Plan* and thank you for doing so.

The following chapters will introduce you to the mechanics of the thyroid gland, how it supports your body, and what occurs when it is not functioning properly. Common problems with the thyroid gland are introduced and explained. Issues, which range from a slight, nonthreatening swelling, to something more insidious such as cancer, are outlined and summarized in a simpler manner. They include a description, list of symptoms, as well as, common treatment methods. Certain individuals are more at risk than others and this book will outline what some of the factors are that can place you at a higher risk, so that you might become more proactive regarding your health.

Food is an important component of maintaining a healthy thyroid and balancing a deficient one. Therefore, the final chapters of this book will focus on diet and the food that you need to consume in order to maintain healthy thyroid. There are certain foods that you should include into your diet, others that you should only consume in moderation and then others that you should completely avoid. A diet plan would not be complete without an easy to follow method and some recipes! Look forward to supporting your thyroid by following the 2-

week diet plan and using the recipes at the conclusion of this book.

There are plenty of books on this subject on the market, thanks again for choosing this one! Every effort was made to ensure it is full of as much useful information as possible, please enjoy!

Chapter 1:
An Overview of Thyroid Problems

The thyroid gland is located in the neck and is an endocrine gland. There are two parts to the gland, which make it appear like a butterfly shape. The two lobes have a central connection called the isthmus, which reaches up to about second ring of the trachea. The thyroid is found under the Adam's apple at the fore of the neck. It binds around and rests against the trachea and larynx. Directly above this gland is the cricoid and thyroid cartilage. The entire gland is encapsulated by a fibrous, thin coating, which has both an inner and outer layer. The exterior layer connects to the cartilage above the gland. This attachment connects the gland to the trachea with a ligament, allowing the gland to motion up and down in order to swallow. The inside layer cuts the tissue into four parts, two for each lobe, and is visible on the backside. Muscles, nerves, and arteries surround the thyroid gland. One muscle is in the front and two muscles rest along its sides. Two arteries run along the back of the gland's lobes. Behind the thyroid are the larynx, trachea, esophagus, and bottom pharynx. Within or next to the ligament attaching the gland to the trachea runs a nerve and an artery.

Several different arteries are responsible for supplying arterial blood to the thyroid. The carotid artery gives blood to the superior thyroid artery and the thyrocervical trunk give blood to the inferior branch. Posterior and anterior branches are split from the superior thyroid artery and directly feed the gland. Inferior and superior branches sprout from the inferior thyroid artery. On the outside and in the back of the gland's lobes the superior and inferior thyroid arteries join each other. Blood from the thyroid's veins goes directly into the jugular vein, amongst other veins. The veins and arteries intersecting between the outer and inner layers of the coating create a complex network.

Synthesis of protein and the rate of metabolism are controlled by the hormones secreted by the thyroid. This is the primary function of the thyroid; however, it also affects a variety of other parts of the body. Some of these functions include:

- *Heart Health:* Your body's blood flow and temperature are controlled by your heart's strength and stability. The hormones secreted by the thyroid increase your heart rate and the power of the muscle. In addition, the hormones deepen your breathing rate, how your body takes in and uses oxygen, and improves the function of the mitochondria.

- *Development:* This is described in more detail below for infants, but hormones from the thyroid also impact child development. T3 and T4 target the cell's in brain development and also encourage a steady growth rate for young children and pre-adolescents.

- *Hormonal Impacts:* The hormones from your thyroid impact your sleeping habits, thought process, and sexual role. When the thyroid's hormones elevated you can think faster but beware, it can negatively impact your focus. For women, your menstrual cycle can be stabilized. For both men and women, your libido can be steadied as well.

Tyrosine and iodine create two hormones in the thyroid, triiodothyronine, or T3, and thyroxine, or T4. Equilibrium of your body's calcium is impacted by another hormone created by the thyroid, calcitonin. An interior pituitary gland releases TSH, or the thyroid-stimulating hormone, which governs the thyroid's output of hormones. This pituitary gland regulates the hypothalamus which produces TRH, or thyrotropin-releasing hormone.

Thyroid hormones need iodine for their production. Iodine, known as iodide when it travels in the blood, is absorbed into cells by a symporter. Once in the cells, iodide deposits ions and leave again, when it leaves it is oxidized into iodine. This process creates a more reactive substance and allows it to bind with other active units, creating the beginning of thyroid hormones. These are then split, and some become the vital thyroid hormones, T3, and T4, amongst others. T3 and T4 are then injected into the bloodstream.

Another hormone that is produced by the thyroid is calcitonin. This assists in calcium regulation in your body. This prevents the bones from breaking down and losing their calcium. It also helps deposit calcium into the bones. If a thyroid is removed or is dysfunctional, calcium absorption and distribution can remain stable because of other hormones in the body, but it does play an impactful role in supporting bone health.

Controlling transcription factors of DNA and hormone reaction components both become bound by hormone receptors from the thyroid. This occurs when cell membranes are crossed by thyroid hormones. Enzyme reactions, like with glucose carriers, occur through thyroid hormones action inside the membranes of cells or cytoplasm.

Women's thyroids are typically larger than men's and the size enlarges during pregnancy. The size and location can vary from person to person. In addition, a third lobe can occur in some people. This is called, "Pyramidal Lobe" or "Lalouette's Pyramid." This is typically a remnant from development. There are other variations of the gland in people, but these are the most common differences.

When a baby is developing, the thyroid is one of the first glands to appear, usually around 4 weeks of gestation. When it first appears, it is located just below the tongue and then begins to descend down the throat to its ultimate resting place just below the Adam's apple in the front of the throat. During its travels it stays connected to the tongue and then, around 5 weeks, it detaches and finally finds its spot. This final, solo travel takes about 2 weeks. The hormones that regulate the thyroid begin to appear in the baby around 11 weeks of gestation. About 19 weeks the baby now has self-sufficient levels of T4. At 30 weeks T3 reaches self-sufficient levels and does not reach full potential until 40 weeks. This development is critical to the overall development of the baby. It protects the baby from neurodevelopment disorders, especially if the mother has a thyroid disorder. The baby must be exposed to proper levels of iodine to reach this full-function.

There are several diseases that could affect the thyroid. Some diseases are a result of too much of a thyroid hormone. This is generally classified as hyperthyroidism. A common hyperthyroid disease is an autoimmune disorder called Grave's disease. Some diseases are the opposite: a result of not enough hormones from the thyroid. This is classified as hypothyroidism. Preventable intellectual disabilities are most often caused by hypothyroidism or iodine deficiency. An autoimmune disorder, Hashimoto's thyroiditis, is the leading cause of hypothyroidism, especially in regions known for iodine deficiency. Other than these two disorders, the gland can also cultivate cancer or nodules. To explain these disorders further, the list below can help you in understanding some of the common issues:

Hyperthyroidism Further Explained:

As explained earlier, when the thyroid creates too many hormones it can create hyperthyroidism. Problems like goiters, inflammation, adenoma, and Grave's disease can cause this to happen in your body. Excess iodine levels can also cause hyperthyroidism from drugs like amiodarone or medical imaging. Hormones that stimulate the thyroid can be overproduced by pituitary adenomas as well. Side effects or symptoms of hyperthyroidism include trouble sleeping, higher sensitivity to hot temperatures, palpitations and tremors, nervousness and anxiety, and unintended weight loss. Other symptoms that are not as common include GI issues like diarrhea, loss of hair, pain in the chest, and weak muscles. Beta-blockers are the common medication used to control these side effects. Thyroid suppressing drugs can be used for more long-term care. In severe cases, thyroid tissue may need to be broken down or completely removed. Completely removing the thyroid does pose certain surgical risks, like disrupting the vocal cords, but it will also result in the opposite problem, hypothyroidism.

Goiter

When your thyroid becomes enlarged and it is abnormal it is labeled a goiter. This is often painless, but it can interfere with your breathing and swallowing. Sometimes the only symptom is a persistent cough or a small lump visible on the outside of your throat. If the goiter is small enough and does not interfere with normal day-to-day functioning, it may be left untreated. Other times it may need medical intervention. The cause of a goiter may be from an iodine deficiency pregnancy, or inflammation, among other problems. For example, another cause could be from many small nodules forming on the gland creating an overall enlargement of the gland. This could be considered either a nodule issue or a goiter issue. Anyone at any time can be affected by a goiter; however, there are some factors that influence this disorder. Women are more susceptible to thyroid disorders in general, which means they are more likely to develop a goiter. Also, if you are over 40 you are more likely to develop a goiter. If you have been exposed to radiation or are taking certain medications, like Lithobid, you could be at greater risk.

Adenoma

An adenoma of the thyroid is typically a follicular adenoma. These types of adenomas are designated as "hot," "Warm," or "cold." An adenoma with a temperature classification indicates that it is a "silent" adenoma. A "hot" adenoma is considered a functional growth and it produces a lot of hormones from the thyroid and may be labeled "toxic thyroid adenoma" because it causes hyperthyroidism. While it may appear to be similar to a goiter, it is distinguished because it is almost always by itself and is a genetic tissue growth from a mutation or abnormality in one cell. To define a growth as an adenoma versus a goiter or a nodule, your doctor must carefully study your thyroid's growth to find its origin and function. Monitoring the adenoma carefully and watching its growth or decline is sometimes all you need to do. Because there are risks associated with an adenoma, you may decide to surgically remove the growth. The risks to consider are interference with normal breathing and swallowing, muscle fatigue, intolerance to hot temperatures, anxiety, irritability, and unexplained weight loss. This is especially true if the adenoma is considered "hot." The other complications include weakened bones, an irregular heartbeat, and an acute attack of increased symptoms, called thyrotoxic crisis. Finally, and adenoma opens up the possibility for the growth to become cancerous. From that diagnosis, there are many additional risks to consider.

Grave's Disease

This autoimmune disease is a result of antibodies being produced that become confused and begin attacking your thyroid gland. This attack results in an increase in a certain thyroid hormone, thyroxine. This overworks the thyroid and makes it swollen. This swelling can be considered a goiter caused by this disorder.

This is the most common cause of hyperthyroidism and the cause of this disorder is unknown. The antibodies that are created typically stimulate the body and create symptoms like weight loss, intolerance for heat, and heart palpitations. Occasionally the symptoms will be more aligned with hypothyroidism because they do not activate the hormone receptors within the thyroid. A unique side effect of this disease also impacts your eyes. In some people, the eyes begin to bulge from the skull and are called Grave's ophthalmopathy. Another swelling may occur in your shins. To treat this disorder, most patients are given a drug to restrict the response of the thyroid, like propylthiouracil. Unfortunately, these drugs are effective but do result in relapse often. If the eyes have been affected, a form of ablation may not be considered, but for all other patients, it is worth considering. Removing the gland can also be a treatment option; however, replacement hormones will be needed, and it will not fix eye or skin symptoms that have occurred in those select patients.

Hypothyroidism Further Explained:

When the thyroid does not produce enough hormones, it results in hypothyroidism. Across the world, iodine deficiency is the leading cause of hypothyroidism. In more developed countries, Hashimoto's thyroiditis is prevalent. Some other less common causes include transient inflammation from various diseases, removal or ablation of the thyroid, various drugs, and genetic abnormalities. Some common side effects or symptoms include heavier menstrual cycles, loss of hair, inability to handle cold temperatures, GI problems such as constipation, fatigue, unintended weight gain, and a slower heart rate. In some cases, myxedema and myxedema coma have occurred, which is a swelling of the skin. A replacement hormone is often prescribed to give your body the necessary hormones and to stifle the symptoms of an under-active thyroid. Sometimes this can be a temporary disorder, such as postpartum or subacute thyroiditis, and other times it can be treated with supplements, like iodine.

Hashimoto's Thyroiditis

This autoimmune disorder can also create a goiter and is similar to Grave's disease in some respect, but it creates the opposite problems. Instead of over stimulating the gland, Hashimoto's hurts the thyroid, so it does not produce enough hormones. Goiters occur when the body senses that not enough hormones are being produced and try to push the damaged gland harder. This stress results in the enlarging of the gland.

This disorder is the most common reason for hypothyroidism in America. Most people that are affected tend to be women and in their mid-40s. In most cases, this disease begins with little to no symptoms and slowly increase over time. Because of this constant damage to your thyroid, the results can be long-lasting. Symptoms patients have reported include fatigue. Intolerance of cold temperatures, constipation, chronically dry skin that is very pale, a swollen face, nails that break easily, loss of hair, a swollen tongue, achy muscles, depression, memory problems and heavy menstrual cycles.

Since women tend to have a higher risk of developing this disease, it is important that she is aware of other contributing risk factors, such as family history of thyroid problems, other autoimmune disorders, and exposure to radiation, particularly around the neck or chest. If someone, male or female, should contract Hashimoto's it can lead to a whole host of issues. For example, an increase in cardiovascular complications, mental health decline, particularly depression and decreased focus, and birth defects. Women who are pregnant and do not have control over their underperforming thyroid have a higher risk for babies with birth defects than those that do not have this autoimmune disease. Birth defects can include physical ones, like problems with the heart or kidneys, and mental.

Nodules

Nodules can be found on the gland surface and are not always cancerous. Sometimes there is a single nodule on the gland and sometimes there are several. Most of the time there are no symptoms of having a nodule. If you have been exposed to radiation, are a female, or are deficient in iodine, it is possible you will develop a nodule or more on your thyroid. If a nodule is detected doctors will test how your thyroid functions to make sure it is producing normally or excessively. If the gland is normal, an ultrasound is used to find out if it is solid or filled with fluid. It will also alert a medical professional if it appears to be malignant or benign cancer. Aspirating the nodule with a small needle may also be required to allow the cells to be examined further under a microscope.

Cancer

Cancer in your thyroid is not as common as benign nodules on the gland. Malignant thyroid cancer is commonly a carcinoma. Very rarely does cancer from another part of the body settle into the thyroid. Women are more likely to get thyroid cancer and radiation on the chest or neck poses a higher risk factor. It is often caught in the early stages of cancer because of the appearance of nodules. The appearance or a mass in the neck, around the location of the thyroid, is often an indication of cancer, especially if the mass is not painful. To treat thyroid cancer, some or the entire gland will be removed. Ablation and radiation may also be an option. When the thyroid is partially or wholly removed thyroid hormone, replacements will be required. This replacement will also hinder the production of TSH, which can cause cancer to reoccur, if not addressed. Most thyroid cancers have a good prognosis and are cured easily. The only exception is anapestic thyroid cancer.

Other Disorders:

Thyroiditis

Thyroiditis is the term used to describe an inflamed thyroid. If a thyroid is inflamed it can cause hyperthyroid or hypothyroid symptoms. Common types of inflammation include Hashimoto's, as described before, or postpartum inflammation. These can show symptoms of hyperthyroidism and then lead to hypothyroidism. Some additional examples of other disorders that can cause inflammation include subacute, acute, silent and Riedel's thyroiditis. Also, palpitation thyroiditis or another traumatic injury can cause inflammation of the gland.

Postpartum Thyroiditis

Postpartum thyroiditis occurs after delivery and is an issue for a period of time before self-regulating and returning to normal functioning. This development can take several months to stabilize and is often identified by the presence of a goiter. Women who have type 1 diabetes at the onset of pregnancy are more likely to have this complication after delivery. Because symptoms are often mild and are known to dissipate after a few months most doctors advise you to wait and watch the abnormality. Medical treatment may not be required; however, during the hypothyroidism stage of this inflammation, some replacement medications may be required. If you do need a medication to help stabilize your hormone you will probably be given a beta-blocker to take for about 1 year postpartum. If you are planning on having many children over the next few years and you had this condition, you should work with your doctor to be on a treatment plan to ensure your thyroid remains stable to support both your own health and the health of the babies.

Congenital

The thyroid's most significant and common congenital problem is an insistent thyroglossal duct. Preemie babies are at a higher risk of hypothyroidism because they did not have enough time to fully develop the glands to meet their post-birth needs. Part of the newborn tests performed in many countries includes checking this proper development. If it is undetected and untreated it can lead to abnormalities in both growth and physical development throughout the child's lifetime. Babies with a low level of thyroid hormones can also have poor mental development. Most children treated for this condition are given a medication to encourage normal development.

Chapter 2:
Who is Affected by Thyroid Problems

General Risk Factors for Thyroid Problems

Thyroid problems have several diseases that you should be aware of. Symptoms may be subtle in the beginning and can be confusing whether you have an under-active or overactive thyroid gland. You may find yourself saying the extra pounds that have appeared may be due to not being as active as usual or your more tired because of stress at work or home. You think they are caused by something else and do not think they are related to a medical issue. Many people admit that the symptoms of a thyroid disorder have been occurring for months and even years before being diagnosed. In general, there are some people that are more at risk of developing a thyroid problem. Some factors are different for different diseases, which will be highlighted later in this chapter; however, this is to first give you a general idea. It is also important to note that thyroid problems are typically not preventable. The best line of defense is to try to live a healthy lifestyle. Change the things you can change, like smoking cigarettes or eating healthier, and accept those things you cannot, like your gender or age.

Here are some general risk factors for thyroid problems:

Being female

It is not for certain why women are more susceptible to developing thyroid issues in their lifetime, but it is clear it is more common. Some theories claim it is because of estrogen and others because women's thyroids tend to be larger than men's making it a larger target in a female's body. It is estimated that women are about 6 times more likely to have a thyroid issue than a male counterpart.

Your Age

For adults over the age of 40, the risk of developing a thyroid problem increases. If a person is over 60 this risk increases further. This is simply due to older age and the body becoming under or over-responsive to the strain being placed on it.

Personal History

Once you have one thyroid problem, it is more likely you will develop it again or another thyroid-related issue. For example, after pregnancy, you had postpartum thyroiditis. Over a few months, it resolved itself. Later on, in life, you are more likely to develop another thyroid problem, like nodules or goiters. Also, if you have another autoimmune disease not related directly to the thyroid, like celiac or arthritis, you are at greater risk. Typically, an existing autoimmune disease, like type 1 diabetes, will lead to a thyroid autoimmune disease, not necessarily cancer or nodules.

Family History

If someone in your close family, like your parents, siblings, or grandparents, has had a thyroid problem, you are more likely to develop an issue yourself. If you are a female and an immediate female member had a thyroid disorder, the risk is even greater. For example, if your mother or sister had a disorder. It can also be an elevated risk factor if you have a daughter that is diagnosed.

Radiation Exposure

You may have received radiation on your neck or chest area for a medical treatment for another disease or reason. For example, if you have cancer in that general area or have Hodgkin's lymphoma, you may have had radiation for a treatment plan. This can sometimes lead to autoimmune disorders in the thyroid and even thyroid cancer. Other times you may have been accidentally exposed to radiation. Similar thyroid problems can occur to those that are exposed to high levels. The people surrounding the Chernobyl nuclear plant when it exploded were exposed to high levels of radiation around them and were at greater risk for thyroid problems, amongst many other problems as well. Sometimes this accidental exposure is not as drastic as a nuclear explosion. If you are undergoing a lot of medical imaging, this constant exposure over time can cause high levels of radiation to affect your body. This is especially true if a medical professional does not prep you properly for the procedures.

Pregnancy and Postpartum

This stage of life for a female poses a minimally higher risk of developing a thyroid disorder. Because many of the symptoms are also attributed to postpartum and pregnancy, it often goes undetected and treated. In the event of a transient disorder, like postpartum thyroiditis, the instability corrects itself after a few months and the body begins functioning again. A postpartum woman has about a 5 percent chance of developing postpartum thyroiditis.

Smoking Cigarettes

Smoking exposes you to a small amount of radiation over time, which can lead to radiation exposure problems. In addition, smoking can increase the risk of developing certain thyroid diseases, including an eye complication from one disease in particular. Not only does it increase the likelihood of developing this disease it also negatively impacts the medication to treat the symptom.

Your Location

If you live in an area that does not have access to iodized salt, you could have a lack of iodine and increase your risk of developing thyroid issues. Since the United States has iodine in most table salts, this is not common in America; however, an increase in salt restriction has become more prevalent over the last several years. If people live in the Midlands or mountains of the United States and restrict their salt it is possible for them to not receive enough iodine. A common recommendation people follow for a "healthier" diet includes changing from iodized salt to sea salt. While this does carry some health benefits, it can cause you to become iodine deficient.

Supplement Intake

If you are sufficient in iodine but take supplements that increase your levels, you also increase a risk for thyroid problems. Sometimes people unknowingly take supplements that have iodine mixed in and other times they take the supplement not understanding the dangers of having too much iodine in the body.

Medical Treatments and Medications

Some drugs and treatments that doctors prescribe may increase the risk of thyroid problems developing. For example, lithium can directly affect the thyroid in many different ways. This is medication to treat bipolar disorders and the risks should be weighed against not taking the medication. Other examples are interleukin-2, amiodarone, and interferon-alpha.

Diet Rich in Goitrogenic Foods

There are certain foods that, especially when eaten raw in large amounts, can increase the risk of thyroid issues. It is important to note that these foods need to be eaten frequently and in large quantities to increase the risk factors. It is because these foods have a chemical in them, called goitrogen, which can increase the risk of a problem and also can interfere with medications for these issues. Foods like broccoli, cauliflower, and broccoli are known to have goitrogen and it is recommended that those who are concerned with thyroid issues should cook the vegetables prior to consuming them.

Diet Rich in Soy Foods

Another food that contains goitrogens is soy. This food source carries different risks than other goitrogenic foods and should be considered on its own. This is because there are conflicting research results on whether there is a direct connection to thyroid disorders or not. It is generally accepted that processed and refined soy products should be avoided. This includes foods made from soy products and soy in pills and capsules.

Traumatic Accidents

Occasionally, when a person experiences a traumatic incident, the body undergoes a tremendous amount of stress. This stress is both emotional and physical. This acute and high-level of stress can overwork the thyroid resulting in thyroid issues.

A final word on general risk factors, some people will develop a thyroid problem with no risk factors. Others will have several risk factors that are relevant to them and never develop a thyroid complication. Risk factors simply increase the likelihood; they do not provide a crystal ball to predict a thyroid disease.

Risk Factors for Specific Thyroid Disorders

There are risk factors that are more associated with certain thyroid issues than others. For example, some risks occur for an overactive thyroid versus an under-active one. Below is a breakdown of who is more at risk for certain thyroid problems.

Surgery on the Thyroid

If you have to have surgery on your thyroid it is typically to remove some or all of it. When this happens, the thyroid cannot generate enough thyroid hormones in your body. It is considered that this automatically results in hypothyroidism or an under-active thyroid.

Received RAI or Radioactive Iodine Treatment

Instead of removing the thyroid in part or in whole this treatment may be used. This is often a treatment for an overactive thyroid, but it results in an underactive thyroid. Someone with Grave's disease or thyroid cancer often receive this type of treatment.

Hyperthyroidism Specific Risk Factors

As described earlier, pregnancies can increase the likelihood of thyroid diseases, specifically hyperthyroidism or an overactive thyroid. Also, having another autoimmune disease, such as type 1 diabetes can result in an overactive thyroid. Finally, having too much iodine is a leading cause of hyperthyroidism. This can be through food or medication; the thyroid does not typically distinguish between the source but rather is trying to adjust to having too much.

Hypothyroidism Specific Risk Factors

Some diseases are the cause of hypothyroidism, directly or indirectly. For example, removing the thyroid or ablating the thyroid can stop overproduction but will result directly in underproduction. Indirectly, your ethnicity may also increase the risk of developing an underactive thyroid. Asian and

Caucasian people have a higher risk factor. Going through female hormonal changes, such as during adolescence and menopause, increases the risk. Also, other disorders such as having bipolar disorder can indirectly cause an underactive thyroid or hypothyroidism. This is because the medication used to treat this issue contains lithium, which is shown to impact the thyroid. Other abnormalities like Turner's syndrome or Down's syndrome can increase the risk factors for hypothyroidism.

Nodule Specific Risk Factors

Nodules can develop for a variety of reasons, both those common for hyperthyroidism and hypothyroidism. For example, having a hypothyroid disorder can develop nodules and personal and family history can impact the likelihood of developing nodules as well. As with many other thyroid disorders, iodine deficiency can also increase the risk of thyroid nodules.

Thyroid Cancer Specific Risk Factors

Some of the risk factors for developing thyroid cancer cannot be changed. These include age, gender, ethnicity, and hereditary conditions. As introduced earlier, women are more likely to develop thyroid issues, including cancer. And people in their mid-40's and older are also more susceptible. Hereditary conditions can be a condition of the thyroid, like an abnormal gene in the thyroid passed down from the parents, called medullary thyroid cancer, or a condition in another part of the body, like colon polyps or colon cancer, can impact the thyroid with benign tumors. Other conditions affect multiple parts of the body, including the thyroid. For example,

Cowden's disease, also known as PTEN Hamartoma Tumor Syndrome or Multiple Hamartoma Syndrome, is a condition where tumors grow throughout the body. There is nothing preventing this disease from developing on the thyroid. Family history also plays a part in increase risk factors.

Some things can be changed and used as a preventative measure for developing thyroid cancer. Not eating enough iodine can result in increased risks of developing certain thyroid cancers. This is especially true if the person is likewise unprotected when presented with radioactivity.

Risk Factors for Children and Infants

Unfortunately, being an infant or child exposed to certain preventable or non-preventable factors can increase the risk of thyroid diseases. For example, radiation and prenatal care can be a high-risk factor. Exposure to radiation at a young age increases the risk factor for developing cancer in the thyroid. This is especially true for radiation centered on the neck or chest area. The younger the child and the higher the dose results in the higher the risk is.

Several decades ago radiation was used as a treatment option for many different ailments that we would not consider today. Ringworm, acne, and swollen adenoids or tonsils are all traditional examples. When children were treated for these non-life-threatening ailments with radiation, it was discovered years later that they had a much greater risk of developing thyroid cancer. Life-threatening diseases like tumors, neuroblastoma, and lymphoma are all childhood cancers treated with radiation also increase the risk of thyroid cancer.

Thyroid cancer developed from other cancers is not any more or less dangerous than other forms of thyroid cancer.

Young children that are constantly exposed to radiation from CT scans or X-rays may also have an increased risk factor. These are often low doses of radiation and it is unclear how more likely a child will develop thyroid cancer than those that do not receive many imaging tests. Despite the uncertainty, it is recommended these tests are only administered when absolutely necessary and when they are they are using the smallest amount of radiation necessary to give a clear image of the child's insides.

Occasionally a child is exposed to high levels of radiation from their environment. This can occur because of radioactive fallout, like when a power plant has an accident or there is a detonation of a nuclear weapon nearby. Adults are also affected, but it is particularly dangerous for children. Those that have enough iodine in their diet before and after being exposed to high levels of environmental radiation had slightly lower risks.

For unborn babies or infants, a mother's thyroid health can be a contributing factor to their risk factors. If a mother has an undiagnosed or untreated thyroid problem she is more likely to miscarry or have a premature baby. Babies also tend to be underweight. The mother can suffer from preeclampsia or a serious increase in blood pressure and congestive heart failure. If the mother has Grave's disease it can occasionally pass to the baby and the infant can begin producing too many hormones. If a baby is born with an overactive thyroid issue the baby can have a quickened heart rate, which may cause their heart to fail. The soft spot on the baby's skull may close too early and it may not gain sufficient weight. The baby may also be increasingly irritable. If the baby's thyroid is enlarged it can make it difficult for the baby to breathe and swallow.

If a mother has an under-active thyroid and passes it on to the baby, the baby may suffer from anemia in addition to a low birth weight and a disrupted heart rate, which could lead to heart failure. Other challenges are related to the mental development of the baby. This is because untreated hypothyroidism does not allow enough hormones to reach the nervous system and brain during development, which happens most critically during the first trimester. These hormones are essential to the cognitive function of a child and if they do not get enough from their mother's during this time they can have a lower IQ and also not developmentally at a normal pace.

Sometimes the risks can be prevented and other times it is uncertain. It is important for mothers to be aware of their thyroid's health while pregnant and work with their doctors to make sure the baby is healthy and receiving the support they need as well. For overactive thyroids, a specialist should be consulted. The medications used are intended to restrict too much of the hormones reaching your baby, but it needs to be monitored closely to make sure enough are still reaching it for proper development. Many forms of hyperthyroidism do not need treatment or medication during pregnancy. Hypothyroidism can be treated with hormone replacement medications to make sure you and the baby receive enough for proper health and development.

Chapter 3:
How to Maintain a Healthy Diet

Thyroid issues affect so many people. It is estimated around 26 million report problems in America alone. Since this little gland is tightly bound to the metabolism, those with these issues can suffer from unintentional gaining or loss of weight. And because it is unintentional and unprovoked, either side effect can be a challenge to address. Weight is not the only side effect to be concerned about. Thyroid problems can lead quickly to other diseases, like diabetes and cardiovascular problems. These are additional reasons why controlling and maintaining a healthy and well-balanced diet are important. Creating a lifestyle centered on healthy choices can enhance your longevity and create a stalemate for some of these problems.

Alone, weight gain can increase the risk of cardiovascular disease, but if someone has a thyroid disorder, the risk is greatly increased. This is because the blood lipid profile becomes higher with thyroid hormone levels lower than average. The lower thyroid hormones also affect blood pressure, inflammation, and amino acid levels by elevating them. LDL or cholesterol levels can also be increased in those with a problem with their thyroid. This is because the glands hormones control the rate of dilapidation, the receptors, and synthesis of cholesterol. Metabolism of carbohydrates is also negatively affected, making it difficult for those with both type 1 and type 2 diabetes to regulate their glucose. Sometimes thyroid problems begin to appear in women around the age of menopause, this is another contributing factor to weight gain, and it can also add to the difficulty of losing unwanted and unprovoked weight gain.

Since weight gain or loss is a side effect of a thyroid disorder, and other problems may exist alongside this issue, it is critical that a dietician is familiar with working with thyroid disorders and how metabolism changes because of it. This will allow them to create goals for you that are achievable, and you can have clear expectations that are feasible. Since the hormones are unstable with a thyroid dysfunction, you should not focus on gaining or losing weight but rather on making healthy choices in your diet and lifestyle. For example, you should focus on eating whole foods, regularly exercising, find ways to relieve stress quickly and get enough sleep consistently. Working with a professional will help you stay focused on these goals and less on the scale. These professionals will also be able to help you find a method for stabilizing your hormones, so you do eventually begin to see the numbers on the scale move.

Creating a meal plan that has a conscious control over the carbohydrates and calories being consumed is essential. The foods in the meal plan should be whole foods and not processed or refined. The focus should be on lean meat, like chicken and turkey, and a lot of vegetables. Include beans and fibers, too. Cutting out or back things like sugar and fats are important, and avoiding fast food is paramount. When eating out, you need to make conscious decisions, trying to choose healthier options. Also, drinking a lot of water throughout the day is important. You should try to drink at least 9 cups of water.

Making these healthy choices leads to possible prevention of other problems and side effects. For example, increasing fiber can help with the side effect of constipation. A healthy diet can also help prevent the development of cancer, diabetes, and cardiovascular disease. All these are connected with thyroid problems and a diet focused on fats that are good for the heart, omega 3, foods high in fiber, and portion control can help manage these risks.

Nutrients

Optimal thyroid function is affected by several diet factors and the symptoms of the disease can be irritated or activated by excessive levels of nutrients or under provided levels of nutrients. This is another reason for working with a professional to stabilize hormone production and control it with diet.

Iodine

Being deficient in Iodine is the world's leading cause of thyroid problems. Iodine makes up thyroid hormones and provides this important nutrient to the body. When it is malfunctioning, it deprives the body of this. Iodized salt led to the reduction of iodine deficiency in America. Other items, such as grains, fish, and dairy, also provide a good dose of iodine in the United States diet. However, much of the salt for Americans now comes from processed foods, which do not use iodine products. This means the iodine intake has slowly decreased and women in their mid-20's to mid-30's typically have a very low intake. Generally, though, American's are still getting enough.

Caution is advised for those who want to supplement with iodine. Having too little carries serious risks just as having too much. For example, too much can cause a flare-up of symptoms for some thyroid problems. It can arouse autoimmune antibodies.

Vitamin D

A lack of vitamin D is common in various thyroid diseases. It is uncertain if the deficiency causes the disease or is caused by it. Regardless of why it occurs, it can help strengthen bones and increase bone mass. This is critical before, during, and after treatment. Bone loss is a common side effect of various thyroid issues.

It is important that you do not go too low or too high with vitamin D, so if you are planning on using supplements, talk with your doctor and allow them to monitor your levels often. In addition to taking supplements, you can increase vitamin D through foods like dairy, eggs, fatty fish, and mushrooms. Sunlight contains vitamin D; however, factors like elevation and seasonality affect the strength of the sun.

Selenium

The thyroid contains the largest concentration of selenium. Selenium is a critical part of enzymes that control the function of the thyroid. Selenium impacts fertility, mortality rates, the immune system, and memory. Having too little selenium can negatively impact the mood and other immune-related functions. Having too much can cause GI problems and increase risks of cancer and type 2 diabetes. A health care professional should monitor your levels of selenium and work with you to stabilize the levels appropriately.

Foods rich in selenium include shellfish like lobster and crab, tuna, and Brazil nuts.

Vitamin B12

The effects of a severe B12 deficiency can be irreversible. It is critical your doctor tests your levels and helps you adjust your intake to be in the correct range. Several people struggling with a thyroid disease can be deficient in B12. Many of the foods that contain high levels of B12 are meat products or by-products, which can make it a struggle for vegans or vegetarians to get enough naturally. Some natural sources vegetarians can eat include nutritional yeast or cereals fortified with vitamins, vitamin B12 specifically. Non-vegetarian sources include fish, like salmon, sardines, and mollusks, and meat from organs, like muscles and liver. Dairy is another good source of vitamin B12.

Goitrogens

Goitrin is a compound that can impede with the combination of hormones produced by the thyroid. It is particularly of concern if someone also has an iodine deficiency. This compound is found in vegetables like cabbage, broccoli, and cauliflower. To modify or remove the effects of this compound you can heat the vegetables. This allows you to absorb the good nutrients while negating the potential negative side effects.

Other goitrogens to be cautious of are soy and millet. Both can impede the thyroid's production of hormones. Soy should be consumed in moderation because the isoflavones can negatively affect the thyroid's hormone production. It does not cause some thyroid problems, but it can exacerbate them. Millet can suppress the function of the thyroid and should be swapped out with another nutritious grain.

Zinc

Having too much Zinc can be considered worse than having not enough. An overabundance of zinc can stop the thyroid from functioning properly. The absorption of copper can be stifled with large doses of zinc and can then lead to a copper deficiency, which is very dangerous. Seeds like pumpkin and sesame are natural sources of zinc, along with food items such as garlic and wheat germ. Foods like dark chocolate and sunflower seeds are especially significant because they are both high in zinc and in copper, helping balance the potential copper deficiency risk with a dose of zinc.

Iron

Enzymes are hindered in their normal activity with a deficiency in iron. Oxygen is deprived of the thyroid with a lack of iron. Adrenals, such as cortisol, are not formed properly and affect the health of the thyroid. Anemia is a form of iron deficiency and can cause a host of problem, including impacting the thyroid. Most notably, anemia negatively impacts the production of red blood cells. However, like many other nutrients, having too much can be negative. The worst-case scenario is toxicity. This can lead to organ failure and even death. Foods high in iron include meats, tofu, fish, and eggs.

Supplements

Taking supplements can interfere with thyroid medications. Because of this, a healthcare professional should be consulted when adding supplements to your daily lifestyle. Timing is critical! For example, Calcium should be taken 4 hours before or after thyroid medication. Fiber can interfere with the absorption of thyroid medications and should be taken 1 hour before or after the medication. This is the same for caffeine, which means coffee should not be used to chase thyroid medicine but rather drunk 1 hour before or after it is taken. Speaking of beverages, be cautious of protein shakes that contain supplements. Some fitness professionals may suggest these shakes to help with increased energy; however, these may interfere with medications because of what is in them. This is especially true if the shake is based with a soy mixture.

Another supplement that is intended for weight loss and glucose control, chromium picolinate, also impacts the ability for medications to be absorbed for thyroid problems. As with a calcium supplement, this should be taken about 4 hours before or after thyroid medication, if someone decides to take it. Flavonoid supplements can also negatively impact the production of thyroid hormones, despite the proven benefits for heart health. Flavonoids from tea, fruits, and vegetables are good sources; however, supplements can have an impact on the function of the thyroid. It is important that you have an open discussion with your doctor if you take or are planning on taking any of these supplements or any others.

Some over-the-counter medications or herbal remedies can interfere with thyroid medication and function. For example, antacids that include magnesium or aluminum hydroxide, like Maalox, should be taken several hours before or after medication. Biotin, another over-the-counter supplement people take for stronger nails or hair can also interfere with thyroid medications when taken in large doses. This means it should be taken in moderation and not within 4 hours before or after taking thyroid medications. Herbal supplements that claim to improve thyroid function can be dangerous due to spiking with drugs and hidden ingredients that are not required to be labeled. Supplements containing kelp can increase hormones that stimulate the thyroid in a negative manner.

While certain drinks and foods may not be a traditional supplement, like tablets or capsules, it is worth noting that some of these items should also be avoided. They can interfere with medication absorption by binding with the medication in the GI tract. Foods to avoid or eat in moderation include items such as walnuts, dietary fiber, flour made from soybeans, and cottonseed meal. In addition to avoiding coffee, as mentioned previously, it is important to also avoid grapefruit juice or at least wait 1 hour before or after medication to consume it.

Exercise

Physical activity is an important factor when discussing thyroid problems and healthy living. Regularly exercising can help with weight management, depression or mood fluctuations, and fatigue. Problems sleeping and experiencing anxiety can also be improved with regular exercise. It has even shown to help some patients to stop taking thyroid medications when they are consistent with their exercise routine.

Just walking and tracking your steps can be a way to increase movement. When you feel fatigued, it can be hard to even think about exercising. Having a tracker or pedometer can be an effective way to monitor your movement but also a way to motivate you to keep moving. Yoga is another method for increasing exercise, especially gentle yoga practices like Hatha yoga, as well as Tai Chi. For those struggling with negative symptoms of a thyroid disorder, strength training and aerobic exercises can also be beneficial. To lessen the impact of strength and aerobic activities, consider water classes like Aquacise. This will help activity be less painful if joints are aching.

Aim for 3 hours of moderate activity per week, if your doctor agrees. Prior to starting your health care, professional may require you to have your thyroid problems under control. Heed their advice and wait for the right time to begin increasing activity. If you do not, exercise could make you feel worse. For example, aching joints may hurt worse or a shortness of breath can be exacerbated during a run or workout. If you do get the all clear to work out more, begin at a slower pace and break as needed. Do not "push through" the pain; stop if you need to. As you become accustomed to the activity level and workouts, increase slowly to take on more and more.

Combining Diet and Exercise

Women are more commonly affected by thyroid issues, probably because of the power of estrogen in the body. Too much estrogen can restrict the function of the thyroid just as too little can strain it. Because estrogen increases and decreases when a woman is in her mid-20's to mid-30's, it is wise to work specifically with doctors to find a balance in hormones by combining healthy eating habits, exercise and environmental exposure, such as to things like pesticides and harmful chemicals, all of which can negatively impact hormone function.

Healthful choices can be hindered by distinctive challenges for thyroid disease such as a change in weight that is unexpected and increased heart risks. Symptoms of thyroid problems like GI upset, fatigue, and mood fluctuations can also impact your desire and willpower to choose healthy behaviors. Aching and sore joints can make physical exercise undesirable. When making changes you need work with your health care professional to focus on heart-centered foods and consistent exercise routines with realistic targets. As you being to reach your goals, both physically and nutritionally, keep working with your health care team to push yourself further in order to fully embrace a healthy lifestyle, and hopefully take full control of your thyroid problems.

Chapter 4:
How to Use Food for Thyroid Problems

There are conflicting reports out there about food good and bad for the thyroid that can be confusing. Some say eat cruciferous vegetables and others that tell you to stay far from them. Below is a compiled list of foods to gravitate towards and a few to truly stay away from. In addition, each item listed includes a reason why you should stay, or you should go. A word of caution, each person is different, and your health care team may suggest you eat or stay away from something listed in this chapter. Please consider their advice prior to trying something below.

Foods to Eat

Brazil Nuts

Selenium is a major nutrient in Brazil nuts. Some thyroid problems should avoid selenium; however, these provide a healthy dose of nutrition and helps convert thyroid hormones and. They also assist in decreasing antibodies in the thyroid. Eat these in moderation to keep your levels steady, no more than 3 per day.

Nuts and Seeds

Nuts, like almonds and cashews, and seeds, like pumpkin and sunflower, are packed with magnesium. This helpful nutrient is critical to the function of a healthy thyroid. Eating them raw, with no added salts or sweeteners can add a crunch to a salad or a great substitute for breading on meats.

Maca

This powerful food contains healthy doses of iron, zinc, and B vitamins. These are all important to a thyroid's proper function. This also helps balance other glands, like the pituitary and hypothalamus, which can help release thyroid hormones and regulate their levels.

Seaweed or Sea Vegetables

Iodine is important for the stabilization of your thyroid. Eating vegetables from the sea helps support proper thyroid function by providing a rich dose of iodine. Nori, hijiki, wakame, and dulse are all examples of sea vegetables. Traditional Asian cuisine has used these ingredients for centuries and many adapted recipes can be found to easily prepare them in delicious foods.

Chlorophyll

This liquid cannot only remove heavy metals in your body that can stop your thyroid from functioning properly, but it can also increase your energy. A small, 1 ounce shot of this can provide a "whammy" of benefits to your day and ultimate health.

Cruciferous Vegetables

Raw cruciferous vegetables can prevent the absorption of iodine because of their high glucosinolates. This could be good if you have to high of iodine; however, many people need iodine in their bodies. For this reason, those with thyroid disorders should eat raw cruciferous vegetables in moderation. This does not mean you have to completely avoid these nutrient-packed vegetables. Consider instead blanching, steaming or wilting the vegetables. Juicing them may also make it easier for your body to absorb the needed nutrients without compromising the thyroid's function.

Leafy Greens

Another good source of magnesium includes leafy greens like kale and spinach. The side effects of low levels of magnesium include irregular heartbeat, muscle spasms and cramps, and lack of energy. These are all controlled by the thyroid, which is directly affected by the levels of magnesium. Other leafy greens include Swiss chard and arugula. It would be difficult to overdo magnesium by using these natural sources, so you can eat several cups per day.

Seafood

Iodine is a critical nutrient for proper thyroid function. Too much and you can have wild mood swings, unexplained anxiety, and an accelerated heart rate. Too little and you face depression, fatigue, and lethargy. Eating a moderate amount of iodine-rich foods can help keep these levels regulated. All varieties of fish, including shellfish like shrimp, are good sources of iodine.

Chicken

The amino acids tyrosine and dopamine are some of the most important elements of the thyroid and its proper function. This is the reason the thyroid responds so well to meats, like chicken. Chicken contains both elements, making it work hard for your thyroid but also for weight management. For example, if you are low on dopamine, you will most likely experience more hunger cues, even if you are not really hungry, and end up gaining more weight. You can find these benefits in foods like dairy and green, too. Thankfully, chicken or other poultry contains these two plus it is lean meat and packs a good dose of B12 vitamins. Both of which give a boost to weight loss and thyroid function.

Salt

Most Americans receive enough salt in their diet, but much of that salt comes from processed foods that contain salt that is not fortified with iodine. Iodized table salt provides a good dose of iodine and is credited for the reason the United States began seeing a decrease in iodine deficiency. While many diets recommend avoiding additional salt intake, some people suffering from thyroid problems that demonstrate a lack of iodine may benefit from adding more of it. Keep in mind that refined foods do not typically contain iodine and neither does sea salt.

Apples

Our bodies can sometimes hold on to heavy metals that are introduced into our bodies. This is because we are not made to process these in high doses. You may be thinking, "But I do not eat metals. This would never be a problem for me." But heavy metals, like Mercury, for example, are found in certain types of fish. Eat too much and you now have high levels coursing through your body, replacing iodine in the binding process and stopping the proper function of your thyroid. Thankfully, some natural solutions are available to help you rid yourself of these metals. Fruits, such as apples, break down into a fiber that has a gelatin-like consistency, called pectin, and it sticks to these metallic compounds, flushing them out from your body. Another perk to this metal-fighting fruit? It also blocks your cells from absorbing as many fat cells, ultimately assisting in weight loss. This pectin is found in other fruits like plums, peaches, oranges, and grapefruits; however, the best pectin is found in whole apples, with the skins still on. This is because it is strongest in the peel and the pit that is fibrous.

Yogurt

Obesity and thyroid issues more often occur when you are low on vitamin D. Yogurt is an excellent source of this essential nutrient and provides a protective barrier for the gland. While you can get a dose of vitamin D from sunshine, aiding with inflammation and improving the immune system, yogurt also contains probiotics, which can help stabilize the gut. A side effect of an improperly functioning thyroid is GI issues, so this may have the added benefit of bringing your tummy to a good place.

Green Tea

Green tea can be an effective coffee replacement and weight loss tool. This is because this magic little drink contains antioxidants called catechins. Catechins tell cells to let go of fat cells and help the liver turn fat cells into energy faster. Since coffee is listed on the "bad" list below, changing it out for this fat-burning liquid could make a big difference in your health and weight goals.

Olive Oil

"Good fats" is a term used to label healthy fats that your body needs and can use to turn food into energy. These assist your body in transmitting the feeling being full, increases your metabolism and shuttle nutrition through the body at increased speeds. Olive oil, particularly extra virgin olive oil, can help achieve all those "healthy fat" benefits but also has shown to improve serotonin within the bloodstream, which aids in the feeling of being full, and a front-line fighter in the battle of cancer, deterioration of the brain, and osteoporosis, thanks to the antioxidants polyphenols contained within the oil.

Eggs

Do not eat just the whites of an egg. While it is true yolks are higher in cholesterol and fats, it contains some of the most beneficial parts, like vitamins and fatty acids critical to boosting the metabolism. Choline is also found in the yolk of eggs, which fights against excess fat stored around your liver. To keep an eye on your cholesterol, do not eat more than 2 whole eggs per day. If you cannot wrap your mind around eating the yellow center, you will still get the benefits of protein in the egg from the whites, while also removing all the fat and lowering the calories in the food, but you will be missing a great weapon in your healthy-lifestyle arsenal.

Whole Milk

Fat is metabolized more quickly because of calcium. Calcium in whole, full-fat milk is abundant. In addition, dairy products help the body eliminate more fat than those who do not eat them on a regular basis. Choose the full-fat or whole versions to up the intake of healthy fats to your diet.

Whole Grain

When the body has to work hard to break down food, it burns more calories. Choosing whole grains means the body has to spend more energy breaking them down. Refined foods, like flour in pasta or bread, are easier for the body to process so it spends less time on them. The body also feels less full of refined foods versus whole grains. Choose whole grains that are also high in fiber, like quinoa, sprouted grains, oatmeal or brown rice.

Garlic

Blood's lipid levels and the metabolism of sugar can be influenced garlic. If a food is known for unhealthy fats and carbohydrates, adding garlic can help them from causing your body harm. Other benefits of garlic include lowered blood pressure, reduction in inflammation, fight cardiovascular disease, and improve the immune system.

Dark Chocolate

Stress, anxiety, and depression are side effects of a dysfunctional thyroid. Many people have unknowingly turned to chocolate to help with stress, but research does support dark chocolate as a method to lower those levels. Dark chocolate also assists in stabilizing metabolism. This is hypothetical because of the flavonoids in the cocoa beans. While it provides wonderful benefits, it is important to note that this is for dark chocolate only, over 70% cocoa, and in small amounts, about 1 ounce.

Beans or Lentils

Lentils, beans, or legumes can contain more than one-third of the required iron intake per day. As little as 1 cup can give you enough to boost your calorie-burning abilities, lower blood pressure, and decrease bad cholesterol.

Kola Nut Tea

Cutting out the coffee can be a challenge, especially for those who enjoy caffeine. Caffeine, if consumed with awareness regarding medication, can help increase metabolism. Choosing a healthy and more effective boost can be found in teas containing this fruit. "Fast Lane" by Celestial Seasonings contains a high dose of caffeine and can help you replace coffee in your caffeine search.

Avocado

Fiber, healthy fats, and antioxidants are all benefits packed into the small, green fruit. The antioxidants kill off free radicals, which are known to kill cells and DNA resulting in all sorts of health problems. While other fruits and vegetables are known to affect free radicals but not like avocados. This amazing food can get to the heart of the free radicals and kill it off unlike anything else. It also makes sure your mitochondria work correctly. This little part helps keep your metabolism working correctly but it can be negatively affected by free radicals; in fact, this is the hub where they congregate the most. Avocados are one of the few food items that can kill off free radicals and support the mitochondria. It is also credited with lowering the risk of various diseases.

Spicy and Sweet Peppers

Both kinds of peppers are known for boosting your metabolism. Many people have heard it is just the hot peppers, like cayenne and chili, because of the capsaicin; however, sweet peppers, like bell and poblano, also supports a strong metabolism because of the dihydrocapsiate. This means no matter your preference for spicy foods, you can use a variety of peppers to support weight loss.

Red Teas

While this form of tea does not contain caffeine, like Kona Nut tea, it does provide wonderful benefits and has a sweet flavor many people enjoy as a replacement for other sugar-based beverages. Besides the delicious taste, red tea, like rooibos, stops new fat cells from forming because of their flavonoids and polyphenols. In addition to stopping fat from being stored, it helps with fat being broken down during the metabolism process.

Bone Broth

Bones contain a large dose of gelatin. When the bones are boiled down into a broth, this gelatin becomes easy to ingest. Once inside, the gelatin helps fill in small tears in your stomach lining, effectively "curing" leaky gut. These tears are dangerous because it allows small pieces of food to get into the blood. Another benefit is the collagen bones provide. Collagen is renowned for improving the strength of your nails, skin, and hair. Protein is also stored in the bones. For those that need to increase their protein but do not want to eat heaping servings of meat, bone broth provides an easy method for delivering it to your body. It is important that you make your own broth or buy it fresh. The "stock" sold in the stores lacks much of the nutrients you are looking for.

Golden Sweet Milk

Mixing almond or cashew milk with honey and turmeric creates a delicious detoxifying drink. It aides your metabolism, fights inflammation, improves your immunity, and helps your digestion. It is creamy and rich and makes a great treat in the afternoon or after a long day!

Ginger Tea

Digestion is improved by ginger. Not only does it help pregnant women with morning sickness, or those affected by motion sickness, but it also calms the GI tract. It helps with issues like IBS and moves foods and nutrients throughout the system at a steady rate. It tells your body that you are full, so you do not overeat, helping people lose weight, and distributes nutrients through the body where they need to go. You can find pre-packaged varieties in the store, or you can make your own by steeping a few slices of ginger root in hot water for a few minutes.

Water

Drink this all day long! Drink a large cup one hour prior to going to sleep. Plain water helps your body detox, give you energy, satiates your appetite, and even helps regulate your digestion. This liquid is vital to your body and it is important to get as much as possible every day.

Foods to Avoid

Meats from Organs

The thyroid can be disrupted when fatty acids are overabundant in the body. In particular, acids like lipoic can lower hormone levels in the thyroid. This is found in high levels within meats like the kidney, heart, and liver of animals. In addition to negatively impacting the thyroid directly, this acid within organ meats can also disrupt thyroid medications. It is for these two reasons you should avoid such meats in your normal diet.

Gluten

Production of antibodies in the thyroid can be stimulated by gluten, especially for certain thyroid problems. Removing gluten can greatly improve thyroid function and hormone levels.

Soy Protein Isolate

Soybeans and fermented soy are not the culprits here. What you should be wary of are the processed soy food items being offered in the stores. For example, alternative "meat" made from soy, soy dairy such as milk and cheese, and granola or energy bars with soy are all refined items from soybeans and can be harmful to your body and especially your thyroid. Be aware of the milk base in protein shakes. Many brands have a soy protein isolate which, again, should be avoided, especially if you have a Thyroid disorder.

Strawberries

Thiourea is a compound found in various fruits, such as strawberries. Similar to raw cruciferous vegetables, this compound can interfere with the thyroids hormone production because it stops iodine from doing its job in the gland. It can create the problems and it can exacerbate them. Limiting fruits that contain this compound, like strawberries, peaches, rutabagas, and pears can help you ensure enough iodine is reaching your thyroid.

Foods Full of "Bad" Fats

A gauge to tell if a food is full of "bad" fat is to recognize your cravings for them. "Bad" fat is highly addictive and has a delicious, but typically unnatural, taste. Grease is another telltale sign of "bad" fat. Foods like pizza, fries, bacon, and burgers are all labeled as "bad" fat foods. They are linked to the feeling of fatigue and reduced energy. They do nothing to help a thyroid problem and often cause or hinder the repair of this vital gland.

Foods Full of Refined Sugar

Refined sugar is found in many American foods. Cookies, soda, candy, and ice cream are all laden with this sweet substance. The rise from a sugar rush is addictive; however, the plummet after the rush is harsh, even more so for those with a thyroid issue. For those suffering from fatigue are hurt most by this rise and fall. If you cannot shake a sweet tooth, choose foods like pitted dates or figs for natural sweetness.

Caffeine

As alluded to earlier, caffeine can counteract thyroid medicines and impact the thyroid. Caffeine, like sugar, can cause an increase in energy and then a harsh crash. This is terrible for those already suffering from fatigue. Also, stimulating your body can overwork your thyroid and confuse it. Coffee is the culprit most people think of when speaking of caffeine. This should be limited to at most 1 cup per day and not with medication; however, soda is a double-edged sword in the healthy lifestyle you are seeking. This drink is not only full of caffeine but also sugar. Soda is best completely eliminated from your diet. If you are craving the bubbles, choose sodium-free soda water with a fresh lemon or lime wedge. The flavor will not be replaced, but your taste buds will change, and your body will thank you!

Processed Food

Extra preservatives and limited nutrients are what you can expect in packaged foods. Any food that comes in a box or a bag that are pre-made should be avoided. This includes packaged chips, crackers, cereals, and cookies. Instead of buying them in a package, try to make them at home so you know what ingredients are in them. Choose recipes with ingredients as close to nature as possible. It may not always be feasible, but it should be something you strive for. As your taste buds adjust to less processed and salty foods the more you will reject them and opt for healthy options.

Chapter 5:
A 14-day Plan and Recipes for a Healthy Thyroid

In an effort to make living with a thyroid problem easier, a simple meal plan is provided below with tasty recipes. The goal is to help you discover what to eat and what to avoid in a realistic way. This is made for busy people at any culinary level and any budget. An additional benefit is that most of the recipes are also gluten-free, which has shown to benefit some different thyroid-related illnesses. Each recipe is full of foods dense in nutrients and vitamins. For example, ingredients contain folate, iodine, zinc, and selenium. Use this plan as a jumpstart to your new lifestyle or pick and choose your preferred recipes and foods to integrate into your diet you are following now. If this is new to you, I highly recommend following this from start to finish to help you stabilize your thyroid and even lose some weight. Two weeks are chosen because it takes that minimum amount of time for your body to adjust to new foods and changes. Just stick with it!

A few recommendations for success include working with your doctor prior to making a major dietary or lifestyle change and leave room for flexibility. The reason for discussing with your doctor is because only you and your medical professionals know your unique needs and history. There are always additional factors, like medications, which need to be considered prior to making any drastic adjustments. In addition, being flexible is important. Some of the recipes may include ingredients you do not eat. Make changes as needed or preferred. For example, if you are following a paleo diet, you may not eat legumes. If this is the case, leave them out or replace them with an alternative that is allowed in the Paleo eating plan. Also, life is busy and sometimes you cannot get into the kitchen to cook up what you want. Plan ahead by preparing some meals and keeping them frozen so you can easily reheat on the go. Other suggestions include choosing water for beverages at meals and throughout the day. You can drink some tea every now and again, but caffeine must be consumed in limitation. Remember, if you are taking hormones for your thyroid, this needs to be taken during a fasting period. This means one or two hours prior to eating you need to take your medicine. Some people prefer to skip breakfast to take their hormones; however, it will depend on your lifestyle and schedule. Decide what works best for you and adjust the meal plan accordingly, if it is necessary.

In the recipes listed at the end of this chapter, many make over two servings. This means you could save the extra serving of leftovers if you are single or double it to feed more. Leftovers are considered in the meal planning so make sure to prepare ahead if you do not plan on having leftovers by the end of the week. If you find yourself without time to cook or need a snack on the go, be mindful of what you grab for. Try to stay away from pre-made foods, junk foods, or processed foods. There is a list of quick snack ideas to consider after the meal plan and before the recipes. It is unrealistic to think you will avoid junk foods or processed foods altogether but be conscious and trying to cut back are important actions to take. The recipes provided will help you make this transition as they are centered on unrefined and whole foods.

The 14-day Thyroid Diet Plan

Monday-Week 1

Breakfast: Green smoothie

Lunch: Gluten-free tuna sandwich

Dinner: Sweet potato skins stuffed with chipotle chicken

Snacks: 1 banana

Tuesday-Week 1

Breakfast: 1 banana

Lunch: Tuna salad made with Greek yogurt

Dinner: Rice and egg shakshuka

Snacks: 1 cup of sliced veggies and either hummus or Greek yogurt for dipping

Wednesday-Week 1

Breakfast: Eggs with sweet potato hash covered with feta

Lunch: Nutty quinoa salad

Dinner: Tasty taco skillet

Snacks: Sweet potato fritters

Thursday-Week 1

Breakfast: eggs served over gluten-free toast

Lunch: Pumpkin soup

Dinner: Sweet potato skins stuffed with chipotle chicken

Snacks: a small handful of Brazil nuts

Friday-Week 1

Breakfast: Chocolate overnight chia seed pudding

Lunch: Middle Eastern inspired salad

Dinner: Leftovers

Snacks: 1 cup of sliced veggies and either hummus or Greek yogurt for dipping

Saturday-Week 1

Breakfast: Green smoothie

Lunch: Tuna salad made with Greek yogurt

Dinner: Eat out or leftovers

Snacks: 1 banana

The Thyroid Diet Plan

Sunday-Week 1

Breakfast: 1 banana

Lunch: Gluten-free tuna sandwich

Dinner: Pesto gluten-free pasta tossed with zucchini and shrimp

Snacks: a small handful of Brazil nuts

Monday-Week 2

Breakfast: Chocolate overnight chia seed pudding

Lunch: Gluten-free tuna sandwich

Dinner: Sweet potato skins stuffed with chipotle chicken

Snacks: 1 banana

Tuesday-Week 2

Breakfast: 1 banana

Lunch: Tuna salad made with Greek yogurt

Dinner: Rice and egg shakshuka

Snacks: 1 cup of sliced veggies and either hummus or Greek yogurt for dipping

Wednesday-Week 2

Breakfast: Eggs with sweet potato hash covered with feta

Lunch: Nutty quinoa salad

Dinner: Tasty taco skillet

Snacks: Sweet potato fritters

Thursday-Week 2

Breakfast: Green smoothie

Lunch: Tuna salad made with Greek yogurt

Dinner: Sweet potato skins stuffed with chipotle chicken

Snacks: a small handful of Brazil nuts

Friday-Week 2

Breakfast: 1 banana

Lunch: Gluten-free tuna sandwich

Dinner: Pesto gluten-free pasta tossed with zucchini and shrimp

Snacks: a small handful of Brazil nuts

The Thyroid Diet Plan

Saturday-Week 2

Breakfast: Green smoothie

Lunch: Tuna salad made with Greek yogurt

Dinner: Eat out or leftovers

Snacks: 1 banana

Sunday-Week 2

Breakfast: Eggs served over gluten-free toast

Lunch: Pumpkin soup

Dinner: Leftovers

Snacks: 1 cup of sliced veggies and either hummus or Greek yogurt for dipping

Snack Suggestions

- Sweet potato chips or wedges

- Fruit and oat balls

- Roasted chickpeas

- Banana bread

- Hummus and veggie sticks

- Peanut butter and greens smoothie

- Chai tea latte with turmeric

- Clafoutis with berries

- Granola-preferably homemade

- Roasted or dehydrated coconut slices

- Goat cheese with figs and gluten-free crackers

Recipes

Below are some recipes, including the recipes for the menu listed above. Experiment, supplement, and have fun in the kitchen!

Breakfast:

Green Smoothie

This recipe needs 5 minutes to prepare and will make 1 serving.

- Protein: 22 grams

- Net Carbs: 24 grams

- Fats: 8 grams

- Calories: 239

- Sugar: 9 grams

- Fiber: 9 grams

What to Use

- Dairy-free milk (1 Cup)

- Chia seeds (1 Tbsp)

- Banana, frozen (1 small)

- Baby spinach (2 Cups)

- Protein powder, vanilla, optional (1 scoop)

- Ice cubes (10)

What to Do

- In a blender, combine all the ingredients and blend until it is smooth.

Eggs with Sweet Potato Hash Sprinkled with Feta

This recipe needs 10 minutes to prepare, 10 minutes to cook and will make 4 servings.

What to Use

- Eggs (4 medium)

- Feta cheese (about 4 Ounces)

- Sweet potatoes, shredded (about 4 cups)

- Extra virgin olive oil (2 Tbsp)

- Baby Spinach, chopped (4 Cups)

- Onion, chopped (1 medium)

- Salt and pepper, optional (as preferred)

- Dried mint, garlic salt, and dried oregano, optional (as preferred)

What to Do

- In a skillet, heat the oil over medium heat and add the sweet potatoes, tossing to cover with the oil. Cook for about 5 minutes, stirring often. Add the onion and cook for another 4 minutes, continuing to stir often. Add the spinach and cook for another 2 minutes, until wilted, continuing to stir often.

- Add seasoning as preferred.

- In the same skillet, make 4 holes in the mixture and crack the eggs into the holes. Cook for about 2 ½ minutes. Cover and cook for another 2 ½ minutes.

- Remove the eggs and hash from the skillet and top with feta crumbles.

Chocolate Chia Seed Overnight Pudding

This recipe needs 15 minutes to prepare, 15 minutes to cook and will make 4 servings.

What to Use

- Dairy-free milk (1 ½ Cups)

- Chia seeds (1/3 Cup)

- Cocoa powder, unsweet (1/4 Cup)

- Sea salt (1/4 tsp)

- Maple syrup (2 Tbsp or as preferred)

- Cinnamon, ground, optional (1/2 tsp)

- Vanilla extract, optional (1/2 tsp)

What to Do

- Combine all the ingredients, except the sweetener, by whisking together in a bowl. Slowly stir in the sweetener.

- Cover the mixture and place in the fridge to cool overnight or at least 5 hours. This will allow the chia seeds to sprout creating the pudding-like consistency.

- This is best when served fresh, but it can last up to 3 days in the fridge.

- Consider topping this with fresh fruit, homemade granola or whipped cream for a different variation.

Breakfast Sausage and Greens

This recipe needs 10 minutes to prepare, 11 minutes to cook and will make 6 servings.

What to Use

- Butter (1 Tbsp)

- Lamb or turkey, ground (1 Lb.)

- Salt (1 tsp)

- Fennel seeds, ground (2 tsp)

- Apple cider vinegar (2 Tbsp)

- Avocado, cut in half (3)

- Mixed greens (6 Cups)

- Olive oil (6 Tbsp)

- Lemon juice, fresh (3 lemons)

What to Do

- In a medium or large bowl, mix the ground meat, salt, fennel, and vinegar until well combined. Adjust the seasoning to your preference. Roll into a log shape and slice into ½ inch thick rounds.

- In a skillet, heat the butter over medium-high heat. Add the sausage and cook for about 6 minutes on one side. Flip and cook another 4 to 5 minutes.

- While cooking, mix the greens with the oil, lemon juice, and salt.

- Divide the greens among the plates, adding sliced avocado on top. When the sausage is done cooking, add it to the plate.

Lunch:

Tuna Salad Made with Greek Yogurt

This recipe needs 10 minutes to prepare and will make 2 servings.

What to Use

- Greek yogurt, plain (1/4 Cup)

- Tuna, canned (5 ounces)

- Mayonnaise (1 Tbsp)

- Apple, diced (1 medium)

- Celery, diced (2 stalks)

- Onion, chopped (1/4 small)

- Garlic salt (1/4 tsp)

- Salt and Pepper (as preferred)

- Lemon juice, fresh (as preferred)

What to Do

- Drain the can of tuna.

- In a large or medium sized bowl, add the apple, celery, tuna, yogurt, and mayonnaise and stir well to combine.

- Stir in the lemon juice and salt and pepper. Adjust the seasoning to your preference.

- Consider eating this on large butter lettuce leaves or gluten-free pita bread.

Middle Eastern Inspired Salad

This recipe needs 5 minutes to prepare and will make 2 servings.

What to Use

- Lemon juice, fresh (1 ½ Tbsp)

- Extra virgin olive oil (1 ½ Tbsp)

- Dijon mustard (1 tsp)

- Honey (1 tsp)

- Salt and pepper (as preferred)

- Bell pepper, red, diced (1/4 Cup)

- Cucumber, diced (1/4 Cup)

- Chickpeas, canned, drained and rinsed (1/2 Cup)

- Quinoa, cooked (1/4 Cup)

- Feta (1/2 ounce)

- Cherry tomatoes, halved (1/3 Cup)

- Olives, minced (2 Tbsp)

- Sunflower seeds (1 ½ Tbsp)

- Baby spinach (1 Cup)

What to Do

- In a small bowl, whisk the lemon juice, olive oil, mustard, honey and salt and pepper.

- In another medium bowl, combine the remaining ingredients. Drizzle the lemon and oil mixture over the salad.

Nutty Quinoa Salad

This recipe needs 5 minutes to prepare and will make 2 servings.

What to Use

- Quinoa, cooked (1 Cup)

- Diced vegetables, any variety (2 Cups)

- Baby spinach, chopped (1 Cup)

- Chopped herbs, any variety (1 Cup)

- Diced fruit, any variety (1 Cup)

- Chopped nuts, any variety (1 ½ Cups)

- Extra virgin olive oil (2 Tbsp)

- Apple cider vinegar (1 Tbsp)

- Lemon juice, fresh (1/2 lemon)

- Honey (1 tsp)

- Dijon mustard (1 tsp)

- Salt and pepper (as preferred)

What to Do

- In a small bowl, whisk the oil, vinegar, lemon juice, mustard, honey and salt and pepper together. Set aside.

- In a medium or large bowl, combine the quinoa with the vegetables, spinach, herbs, and fruit. Drizzle the oil and vinegar dressing over top.

- Top with chopped nuts.

Pumpkin Soup

This recipe needs 5 minutes to prepare, 25 minutes to cook and will make 8 servings.

What to Use

- Pumpkin, canned (2 Cups)

- Onions, whole, skins removed (2 medium)

- Garlic, whole bundle, skin removed (1 medium)

- Vegetable stock (6 ¼ Cups)

- Salt and pepper (as preferred)

- Barley, pre-soaked overnight (1 Cup)

- Quinoa, not cooked (1 Cup)

- Chia seeds (1/2 Cup)

What to Do

- In a large saucepan, combine the pumpkin, onion, garlic, and stock. Bring to a boil for 5 minutes.

- Using an immersion or hand blender, blend until smooth.

- In another saucepan, combine the barley and quinoa with required water and boil for 15 minutes. Drain the mixture.

- Stir the quinoa and barley mixture into the pumpkin puree.

- Stir the chia seeds into the pumpkin and quinoa/barley mixture.

- Bring the soup to a boil and boil for 5 minutes.

- For a smoother texture, use an immersion or hand blender or serve it as is.

Dinner:

Sweet Potato Skins Stuffed with Chipotle Chicken

This recipe needs 15 minutes to prepare, 1 hour 20 minutes to cook and will make 8 servings.

What to Use

- Sweet potatoes (2 medium)

- Chicken breast, boneless and skinless (3/4 lbs.)

- Extra virgin olive oil (1/4 Cup)

- Lime juice, fresh (2 Tbsp)

- Garlic, minced (2 cloves)

- Chipotle peppers, minced (3 whole)

- Oregano, dry (1 tsp)

- Cumin (1 tsp)

- Chili powder (2 tsp)

- Salt and pepper (as preferred)

- Baby spinach (2 Cups)

- Cheddar cheese, shredded (5 ounces)

What to Do

- Preheat the oven to 350 degrees.

- Wash and prepare sweet potatoes to be baked by pricking with a fork. Bake for about 50 minutes.

- In a baking dish, place the chicken breasts and rub with olive oil and salt and pepper, as preferred. Bake for the final 25 minutes of the sweet potatoes.

- Shred the chicken when cooled. Halve the sweet potatoes and cool for 10 minutes.

- Combine the olive oil, lime juice, peppers, garlic, herbs, and salt and pepper in a medium or large bowl.

- In the microwave or on the stovetop, wilt the spinach quickly. Stir into the shredded chicken.

- Increase the oven temperature to 400 degrees.

- Scoop out the insides of the sweet potatoes, leaving enough flesh to keep the skins strong. Use the insides for another recipe.

- In a new baking dish, place the skins inside and lightly cover with the chipotle sauce. Bake for 10 minutes.

- While baking, combine the remaining chipotle sauce with the spinach and chicken mixture.

- When the skins are done baking for 5 minutes, stuff them with the chicken mixture and top with the shredded cheese. Bake for another 10 minutes.

Rice and Egg Shakshuka

This recipe needs 10 minutes to prepare, 35 minutes to cook and will make 4 servings.

What to Use

- Extra virgin olive oil (1 Tbsp)

- Garlic, minced (1 clove)

- Onion, diced (1 medium)

- Bell pepper, diced (1 medium)

- Plum tomatoes, whole and peeled (1 can)

- Paprika (1 tsp)

- Jalapeno pepper, pickled and chopped (2 pieces)

- Eggs (4)

- Rice, uncooked (1 Cup)

- Water (2 Cups)

What to Do

- In a skillet, heat the oil over medium heat. Sauté the garlic, onion, and pepper for about 5 minutes.

- Stir in the tomatoes and the juice from the can, paprika, and peppers. Break apart the tomatoes gently. Simmer for 25 minutes.

- While the sauce is simmering, cook rice in the water according to the directions, typically about 5 to 10 minutes.

- Add the eggs on top of the tomato mixture and cook for about 3 minutes until the whites are cooked and the yolk is hard but not cooked all the way through.

- Using a spoon, place an egg on a plate, add about ¼ of the rice to the plate, and cover with the tomato mixture.

Pesto gluten-free Pasta tossed with Shrimp and Zucchini

This recipe needs 5 minutes to prepare, 10 minutes to cook and will make 2 servings.

What to Use

- Shrimp, peeled (1/2 lbs.)

- Gluten-free angel hair pasta, cooked (4 ounces)

- Zucchini, chopped (1 small)

- Bell pepper, chopped (1 medium)

- Pesto sauce (1/3 Cup)

- Extra virgin olive oil (2 Tbsp)

What to Do

- In a skillet, heat ½ of the olive oil over medium-high heat and add the shrimp. Do not stir so they brown and get a crunchy layer. Remove and set aside.

- Add the last ½ of the oil, peppers, and zucchini to the skillet and cook for about 4 minutes, until cooked through.

- In a medium bowl, place the cooked pasta, shrimp, pepper and zucchini mix, and the sauce. Stir to combine.

Tasty Taco Skillet

This recipe needs 5 minutes to prepare, 15 minutes to cook and will make 6 servings.

What to Use

- Ground beef or turkey (1 lbs.)

- Onion, diced (1 medium)

- Bell peppers, diced (2 medium)

- Tomatoes with green chilis, diced (1 can)

- Zucchini, diced (2 large)

- Baby spinach (3 Cups)

- Cheddar cheese, shredded (1 ½ Cups)

- Chili powder (1 Tbsp)

- Cumin, ground (1 tsp)

- Garlic powder (1 tsp)

- Paprika (1 tsp)

- Oregano, dried (1/2 tsp)

- Onion powder (1/2 tsp)

- Salt (1/4 tsp)

- Pepper (1/4 tsp)

- Red pepper flakes, optional (1/4 tsp)

What to Do

- Mix all the seasonings in a small bowl. Set aside.

- Brown the meat in a skillet over medium-high heat. Remove the liquid fat.

- Add the onion, pepper, and zucchini and cook through.

- Add the tomatoes and seasoning. Stir to combine.

- Add the spinach and stir in to wilt.

- Top with the cheese, cover, and allow to melt over the top for about 5 minutes.

Snacks:

Sweet Potato Chips

This recipe needs 10 minutes to prepare, not including the 1 hour of soaking, 2 hours to cook and will make 5 servings.

What to Use

- Sweet potatoes, sliced evenly (2 medium or large)

- Extra virgin olive oil (2 Tbsp)

- Salt and pepper (as preferred)

What to Do

- Place the sliced potatoes in a bowl of cool water to soak for 1 hour. Pat dry.

- Preheat the oven to 250 degrees.

- In a medium bowl, toss lightly the potato slices with the oil and spices, as desired.

- On a baking pan, layer the potato slices evenly across.

- Bake the chips for 1 hour, then flip them and bake for another hour. Allow to cool for 10 minutes before eating.

Fruit and Oat Balls

This recipe needs 10 minutes to prepare, 1 hour to cook and will make 8 servings.

What to Use

- Dates, pitted (10)

- Almonds, raw (1/4 Cup)

- Cashews, raw (1/4 Cup)

- Blueberries, frozen (13 Cup)

- Vanilla extract (1 tsp)

- Nut butter (1 Tbsp)

- Coconut, shredded and unsweet (as preferred)

What to Do

- In a food processor or blender, process the dates, nuts, nut butter, and extract until combined and chunky.

- Add the blueberries and process until combined.

- With wet hands, create balls with the mixture and freeze for at least 1 hour.

- In a medium bowl, place the coconut. When the balls are frozen for 1 hour, roll them in the coconut to coat. Keep in the fridge or freezer.

Conclusion

Thank for making it through to the end of *The Thyroid Diet Plan*, let's hope it was informative and able to provide you with all of the tools you need to achieve your goals whatever they may be.

The next step is to start making the positive changes that you can make. Do this to decrease your risk factors for developing a thyroid disease or to help your body find homeostasis if you are experiencing a thyroid problem already. Work with your doctors and medical team to determine your thyroid risk factors, and how to treat a current condition. Part of the conversation should include your diet. Work with them on how to integrate good food choices into your daily routine to support your body, no matter if you have a thyroid problem already or not.

Not every person who has risk factors will develop a thyroid problem and some people will never show a risk prior to having a thyroid issue. In addition, some risk factors are not controllable. Most of the time thyroid issues cannot be prevented. The best you can do, no matter the state of your thyroid, is to be vigilant and make good choices. The recipes and the diet plan provided in this book are a guide to get you there. Good luck! And remember, any small change to positively support your body and thyroid is not for nothing!

Finally, if you found this book useful in any way, a review on Amazon is always appreciated!

www.ingramcontent.com/pod-product-compliance
Lightning Source LLC
Chambersburg PA
CBHW070027260726